Speed Strong

Speed Strong

By
Josh Bryant and Adam Benshea

Introduction

One of the most deflating experiences is to find yourself living a life void of purpose.

Conversely, one of the most fulfilling experiences is living a life filled with purpose.

Now, filling the vessel of your life with the cargo of purpose can be an arduous task. For this reason, we provided you, our readers, with works to get your mindset in order (refer to *Jailhouse Strong: The Successful Mindset Manifesto* and *Grounded in Gratitude: A Call to Action*). Of course, you may be pursuing a wide array of paths, projects, and purposes.

However, a singular drive unites all of our readers: the pursuit of strength. In this quest, strength is the goal, but it is also a necessary companion for the attainment of any worthy objective. Whether you want to climb the corporate ladder, hit a new PR on the bench, or finally make the first team of the male revue at your local casino, you need strength of both an emotional and physical quality.

Every one of our books, programs, and training guides is written with the intent of you becoming strong and staying strong. As a matter of fact, the strength to endure is one of the most difficult, but crucial, components for any individual who is carving their course through a purposeful life.

The Russian playwright Anton Chekhov once wrote: "Any fool can survive a crisis. It's the day-to-day living that wears you out."

Many can rise to an occasion. Few can rise out of bed every morning to slog onward in the pursuit of a goal that is blocked by a seemingly endless line of obstacles which can only be traversed through activities that are extraordinary because of their previously unfathomable monotony.

Nonetheless, you keep moving forward. You keep moving forward, with strength.

Martin Luther King Jr. once said: "If you can't fly, then run, if you can't run, then walk, if you can't walk, then crawl, but whatever you do, you have to keep moving forward."

Yet, some strength athletes, tactical athletes, and combat athletes who have been in the arena for many years become limited in their movement options because they have become locked in repetitive patterns of activity.

The definition of failure is failing to realize that you still have a choice—a choice to improve and escape your current predicament. The definition of success may be nebulous and individualistic, but it is related to having more choices rather than fewer.

To broaden your movement options, to give yourself more choice in the expression, attainment, and preservation of your strength, you need to be able to move with speed and strength.

You need to become speed strong.

Let's talk about what we learned and how you can attain it.

Fast-Twitch Muscle Fibers

You must believe in yourself to make something of yourself. While that may sound trite, it doesn't make it any less true. And, like any truth, you must experience it to know it.

The journey to the attainment of self-affirmation can get a powerful boost when someone else believes in you, when they say you matter.

Knowing we matter is crucial for any of us at any time, but it is particularly poignant during that formative period of adolescence. Perhaps one of the most self-affirming experiences is the confidence gained through athletics. With dedication and discipline, a young person can watch an almost mystical transformation of character through the acquisition of strength and skill.

Certainly, that was the case in our experience. From our determined efforts, our bodies became hard and our hands became skilled in the arts of contact sports. Thereafter, we got noticed. Girls turned their heads in our direction (perhaps not as many as we would have liked). School administrators gave us praise.

We would also receive compliments from many of the old-timers in the community. You know, the guys who skip social media updates to still read the sports page of the local newspaper. One such individual was Al Torrio. He had kids who attended the private school in our town and achieved athletic acclaim in their own right. Although they had since graduated, Al continued to follow sports and liked to be involved in high school athletics.

As we wrote about in our book *The Saga of the Tijuana Barbell Club*, we grew up in a small beach town. Now, in the sprawling hills behind our community, there were a growing number of premier wineries. In the midst of these estates, which were more snooty and refined than bacchanalian and rowdy, Al had a horse ranch.

The stories that came down from the hills about his ranch were epic. He would hold parties for league championship teams. Nothing sinister or out of control, just some old-school fun. You know, real backwoods stuff. ATVs, skeet shooting, hog hunting, and even some catfish noodling (before the time-honored method of fishing became a viral sensation on the internet).

So, we had this on our minds the day we ran into Al, as we walked out of the gym. He was wearing his trademark tank top, which revealed a broad chest and powerful shoulders, and old-school shorts, which showed his thick upper legs. All the big muscle groups were clearly developed.

"Hey, I know that thousand-yard stare. You guys just finished up some hard training. Man, you boys don't mess around."

We attempted to brush off his compliment.

"You can't hustle me, I've been to the shadiest of Detroit pool halls and came out on top."

Not sure how to respond, we gave a slight chuckle.

"Hey, enough small talk, I got to hit some shoulders," he said while shrugging his broad delts for effect. "Yeah, fellas, I'm having some people up at my place this weekend, some coaches and a few trainers. It would be great to have you guys there. I'll have my secretary get you guys the details.

"All right, time to hit the gym," he said, without waiting for us to respond. He nodded brusquely and rushed on to his workout.

So, after a call from his secretary (who had a voice like dripping honey), that next weekend we found ourselves pulling up to Al's Tuscan-style palatial estate.

As we stepped into his foyer, we noticed the high beam ceiling, ornate chandelier, and marble floor, which made the house look like something from a gangster movie. This wasn't surprising, given the rumor that Al was a connected guy (meaning he had associations with some of the "families" back east).

Before our imagination could get the better of us, Al came to greet us with a broad smile.

"Fellas, I am so glad you could make it. Come out back, everyone is out by the BBQ pit," he said, making a broad stroke with his massive arm. A simple wave of the hand would have been too dainty for Al. There was nothing dainty about Al.

Following him out back, we saw an expansive setting of a lush garden and stables framing one of the most elaborate BBQ setups we had ever seen. Sitting around a large spit of meat rotating over a massive bed was a motley crew of local physical cultural legends—some we knew and some we just knew of.

There was Coach Chiefy (from *Jailhouse Strong: 8 x 8 Offseason Powerlifting Program*), the mystical Rocky

Now that you are "woke" (i.e., alert to injustice in society, or, in this instance, the gym), you should start to question antiquated, outdated modes of training authority. It makes you wonder.

First question: Why are fast-twitch fibers neglected in aesthetic-driven training programs?

Next question: Why do tactical athletes think that bastardized renditions of Power Clean AMRAPs will work fast-twitch fibers?

This type of self-delusion is comparable to the tripped-out hippies who attempted to levitate the pentagon (with a goal of 300 feet off the ground) in a communal acid trip war protest in 1967 (the pentagon is still there, if you are wondering).

To start answering these pressing questions, let's process some information.

Okay, your body is outfitted with a mixture of muscle-fiber types that exist on a continuum. The spectrum spans from smaller, endurance-based, slow-twitch fibers to large fast-twitch fibers designed for speed, strength, and power.

Large in size, fast-twitch fibers store large amounts of carbohydrates. In fact, each stored gram of carbohydrate draws approximately three grams of water into the muscle. This is part of the reason why bodybuilders who lift heavy, and conversely maximize fast-twitch fiber, look fuller and dense.

And while our training program will make you more Gas Station Ready (that is, tactically competent and functionally capable), the program also invokes the growth of fast-twitch fibers which will make you Chippendales Ready (that is, aesthetically pleasing to the scantily clad attendees at your neighborhood pool party).

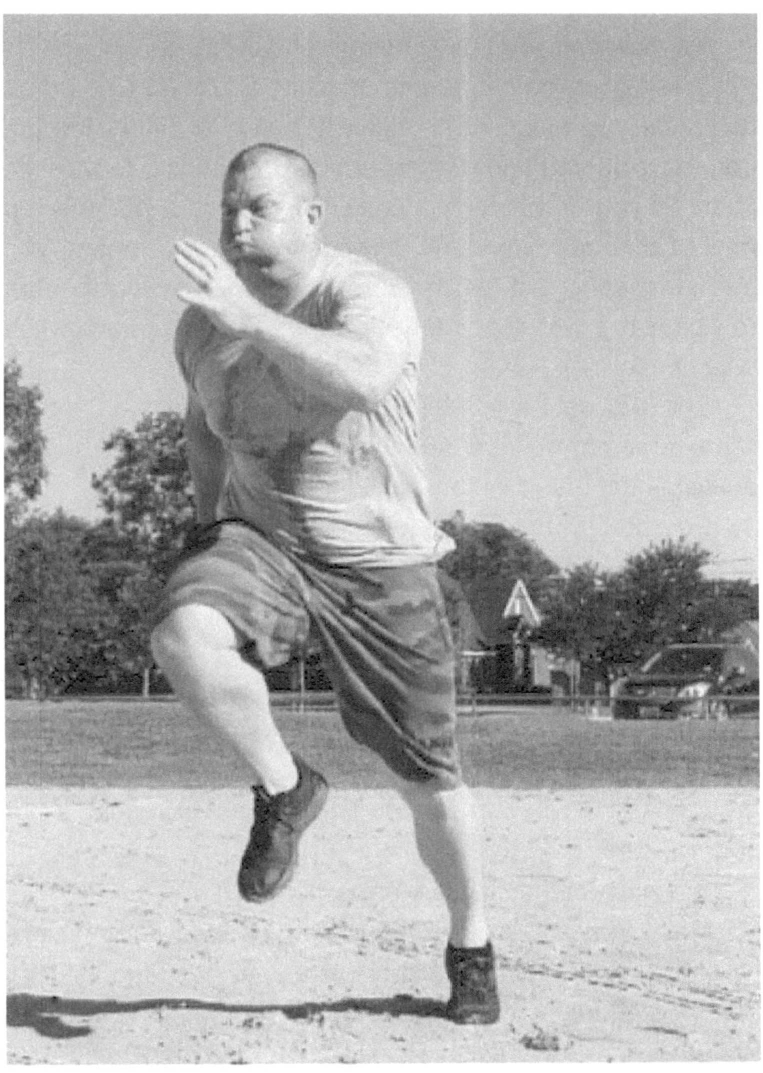

Fast-Twitch Recruitment

All right, so you're on board with the #GASSTATIONREADY movement, and you would like to look #CHIPPENDALES-READY.

So, how can you recruit fast-twitch fibers?

Well, your body recruits muscle fibers by the force demands you place on it. So, when you're hitting the pig iron, how do you know whether you are training fast-twitch fibers? If you lift with high intensity in relation to your one-rep max of a large, compound, strength-based movement, you are hammering fast-twitch fibers. In contrast, going through rep after rep with low intensity keeps you in a slow-twitch safe space.

The lab coats in a 2004 study demonstrated that Olympic lifters and powerlifters had much greater fast-twitch fiber development than their bodybuilder brethren.

For the Olympic lifters, it is not surprising that they have significant fast-twitch fiber development because they move weights in very fast, athletic, triple extension movements. Although powerlifters move heavy weights slowly, fast-twitch adaptations are imposed from the heavy weight lifted in the one- to five-rep range, with long rest periods. Now, with the high rep and short rest period training of many bodybuilding programs, their greater slow-twitch fiber development is not surprising.

So, why do bodybuilders have more muscle?

Mainly drugs. Secondly, nutrition and slow-twitch development are necessary to fully develop a physique, and this can easily be remedied with added "pump work" (i.e., higher reps more traditionally associated with bodybuilding). Because of this fast-twitch stimulus, the bodybuilders who have not yet trained with a fast-twitch focus can expect to add slabs of muscle mass.

Aside from heavy lifting, explosive, high-force movements that require ample rates of force development recruit fast-twitch muscle fibers. The two best examples are sprinting and jumping. While both are used in our program, sprinting is the primary driver.

We have written extensively about the benefits of strength training, and we have written some about sprinting. Let's develop the latter a little and learn how sprinting will help you chase down criminal suspects, improve your game on Tinder, enhance your physical health, sharpen your mental acuity, and balance your emotional well-being.

Sprinting

Sprinting is the most versatile form of exercise because it is utilized to build power and speed, increase muscle hypertrophy, shred body fat, and increase your cardiovascular capacity and muscular endurance. No other singular form of exercise can match this.

Legendary late strength coach Charles Poliquin used to say, "Do sprints to lose fat, build muscle, improve your health, and live a more excellent life. Sprint training is a powerful tool that gives you back considerably more in terms of health benefits than the effort required."

Here is a quick overview of what sprinting can do for you.

1. **Reduce body fat.** Multiple scientific studies confirm sprints are superior to steady-state cardio for fat loss and are much more time efficient. Anecdotes close the case—skinny-fat distance runners don't look as good in their three-piece suits or birthday suits as sprinters! Some studies show sprint programs can reduce the body fat of participants by 10 to 20 percent over 12 weeks.

2. **Build muscle and target fast-twitch fibers.** Studies show sprinting can enhance muscle protein synthesis by more than 200 percent while building your fast-twitch muscle fibers. Assuming nutrition is dialed in—and if it's not, start (with *Nutrition, Your Way*)—this will build a lean, more muscular physique that is not just smoke and mirrors.

3. **Increase hormonal response.** For men, repeated sprints will flood you naturally with a cascade of anabolic hormones (testosterone and growth hormone), meaning you will be waking up stiff—and we are not talking about decrepit, but pitch-a-tent stiff! Ladies, because you won't experience the same testosterone boost, you don't have to worry about matching your man's beard, but the sprints will increase growth hormone levels, producing a sexy, strong feminine outcome that will catch the eye of the tall, dark, and handsome, independently wealthy guy who just got an office down the hall.

4. **Increase work capacity.** Strength athletes and traditional athletes alike benefit from work capacity gained through sprinting. Repeated sprints result in more efficient energy utilization by increasing the amount of glycogen that can be stored in a muscle by approximately 20 percent (giving your muscles that dense, full look). Plus, repeated sprints train the body to become more effective at removing waste products during exercise, greatly increasing the muscles' buffering capacity. Because you are now faster from sprinting, your submaximal zone is higher; your 70 percent of max speed is higher than most untrained people's 100 percent.

5. **Increase time efficiency.** Sprinting means going all out; you cannot go all out for hours on end. This makes sprinting very time efficient; that is why the volume of the program, at first glance, seems low. Nasty, brutish, and short, paraphrasing Thomas Hobbes, is all we need.

6. **Increase mental toughness.** Sprinting ain't for limp dicks, it's hard! Sprints hurt. You will be in pain and question if it's worth it during these workouts, assuming you give 100 percent. Persevere! You got this. Focus on the pleasure you will achieve both physically and mentally by completing this program, not on the pain of the individual sessions. Performance, health, aesthetics, and vitality will prevail when you see this through.

7. **Improve lung function, heart health, and circulation.** In some studies, those who did sprints showed greater improved lung capacity compared to those who did aerobic training protocols! Furthermore, sprint protocols have been shown to decrease blood pressure and cholesterol and improve circulation.

8. **Improve brain function and help to prevent depression.** Almost all forms of exercise improve brain function; if this subject interests you, read the book *Spark: The Revolutionary New Science of Exercise and the Brain* by John J. Ratey, MD. Sprint training appears to be the Taj Mahal of exercises because it decreases inflammation in the brain, increases mobility, escalates energy levels, and improves hormonal balance.

9. **Build stage-ready muscles.** "Old men have pancake asses because they don't sprint!" So said the legendary Al Vermeil. In bodybuilding, striated glutes are now the standard. On the bikini stage, shows are won

you cannot just do one or the other to get the intended training effect of our program.

In particular, let's look at sprints and heavy squats. Both recruit fast-twitch muscle fibers, but they do so in a different fashion. When you're sprinting, the negative (eccentric contraction) is ballistic; with squatting, the eccentric is very controlled, even with an efficient dive bomb technique.

With sprinting, there is a huge reliance on the stretch reflex (think rubber band–like effect); with squatting, there is a reliance on the stretch reflex but not nearly to the extent of a sprint, even with a rapid descent. This is because the descent on a squat is at a predetermined and controlled pace, while a sprint is cyclical in nature and is at full speed.

Strength coaches rightfully advocate lifting explosively. Regardless of the intent to perform a movement with maximum acceleration, the positive (concentric) portion of the lift is much slower than a sprint.

With squatting, the load remains constant; 400 pounds is 400 pounds. While more effort will be required in the bottom portion, you are still lifting 400 pounds (plus your bodyweight). With sprinting, your bodyweight will be magnified by four to six times, depending on the strides you are taking.

Mechanics

Unless something is *way* off technically, you will receive benefits from sprinting. This is not a manual on sprint technique, but, still, we will do a quick review of sprint mechanics.

When it comes to sprint speed, the two most important factors are stride length and frequency. Now, there are two fundamental segments of speed and acceleration, and they differ in function and body position. The two segments are the transitional phase and top speed. As you accelerate, there is a transitional phase to reach top speed. After top speed is reached, your objective is to maintain it for as long as possible. For Olympic sprinters, top speed is reached at 50 to 60 meters and it can be maintained for an additional 10 to 30 meters.

When accelerating, remember to drive out at a 45-degree angle from the ground while you push into the ground with each sequential step. A 45-degree angle facilitates force generation so that when the foot hits the ground, it will instantaneously explode off it. This improves force output and increases stride length.

After you transition to where you are running at maximal speed, you should shift vertically between 80 and 85 degrees from the ground. From this position, you will be pulling your leg back as your foot strikes the ground. This will optimize your stride length.

Further Sprint Mechanics Guidelines

Arms and Shoulders
- Your arms should be moving front to back in a fast, smooth motion; avoid crossing your body.
- Extend your fingers out. Clenching your fists wastes energy.
- Your arm movements should be in balance with your leg motions.
- Your hands should be level with your chin. From here, throw your hand down as forcefully as possible. Then drive back as far as possible.
- Keep your shoulders relaxed and low, not clenched or shrugged.

Posture

- Your trunk should be at a neutral angle, not leaning forward or backward.
- Think of your posture as a straight line from your head down through your hips and the balls of your feet.
- Your hips should be aligned so they are facing straight ahead.
- Relax your facial muscles and neck while keeping your head straight. Look forward and slightly down.

The goal is not to get you ready for the Olympics; while you will benefit from this program with suboptimal sprint technique, you can maximize your benefits by following the guidelines above.

Putting It All Together

Again, both heavy lifting and high-speed activities torch fast-twitch fibers. But, as George Washington Duke says in *Rocky V*, "Timing is the essence of life."

Timing and dosage are everything, whether it's a recipe for seafood gumbo, a head butt in a bar fight, or a great training plan.

Through real-world trial and error combined with sound scientific principles, we have taken the guesswork out of the equation.

Remember, success leaves clues. Look at the physiques of top-level sprinters, whether it's Ben Johnson or Harry Aikines-Aryeetey. Or, hey, just go to a high-level track meet and watch a 100- or 60-meter sprinter. These guys are jacked, often more so than competitive natural bodybuilders or those wannabe bodybuilders at LA Fitness.

So, why do these sprinters have bodies that most supplement-swallowing gym rats only dream of?

Partially because their muscle has a much denser look. This is due to sprinters possessing a higher concentration of contractile muscle. This is noticeably different from gym bodybuilders who only train for a pump, which can be easily deflated.

The reason Ronnie Coleman, Dorian Yates, and Branch Warren are pumped while also looking strong is because they come from a strength background. They train hard and have built up contractile muscle fibers. The aforementioned bodybuilders' look of "density" is a result of myogenic tone.

Myogenic tone refers to a state of partial muscle activation. Myogenic tone means that, even at rest, the nervous system keeps some tension on the muscle. Because the muscle is partially activated, it can and will be ready to instantaneously produce force, if needed. To develop this, the muscle looks like it's in a partial state of contraction, as opposed to a muscle looking like a balloon filled up with air.

So the way in which Dorian, Ronnie, and Branch separate themselves from the crowd can be attributed to the same factor that causes sprinters to be built like brick shit houses—myogenic tone.

For the most part, myogenic tone results from two mechanisms.

Neural efficiency: The more efficient your nervous system, the greater your myogenic tone will be. Sprinting improves the neural aspect of running much more than a Kenneth Cooper inspired, testosterone-robbing jog; heavy lifting is superior to light lifting for improving the neural aspect of force production.

Fast-twitch fiber development: Research has shown that fast-twist fibers are more superficial (closer to the skin surface), in contrast to slow-twitch fibers deeper in the muscle. By developing fibers closer to the surface, your muscles aesthetically have a more solid/dense look. This effect is amplified with a low percentage of body fat.

This is why the physiques of pump and pose fluffers look different from those of real lifters.

Another, often overlooked, aspect of myogenic tone is timing.

Admittedly, 15 minutes into a workout, a fluffer will look much more impressive than when he's in a relaxed state, but catch him two hours after training, and he deflates back to normal. An athlete with myogenic tone does not have these fluctuations.

With this program, you are going to maximize fast-twitch fiber recruitment in a way that will produce the look with the firepower that *should* follow.

You'll be looking #chippendalesready while staying #GASSTATIONREADY.

You are going to do this by overloading your nervous system with a heavy strength-training movement. Then, immediately after, you are going to have to generate the power while fatigued to produce top speed.

You will be taxing your fast-twitch fibers with high-force, low-velocity strength-training movements, then, at the drop of a hat, bursting into an explosive, high-force, high-speed contraction. We will tax the spectrum of fast-twitch fibers with a low-speed and a high-speed activity that will produce a magical synergy.

This particular program was inspired by Ben Johnson squatting 500 for five reps, then immediately bursting out of the rack into an all-out 60-meter sprint.

Beyond the benefits and the reasoning of why this works that we've already described, here are some more considerations.

Now, some of you may be familiar with the concept of post-activation potentiation (PAP), which is the theory that an intense movement performed before an explosive activity can increase power. With this in mind, why not wait five-plus minutes for a PAP effect?

Well, the conditioning and some of the hypertrophic benefits would be compromised. By keeping rest intervals shorter (but long enough to sprint at nearly top speed), you are taxing the fast-twitch fibers in their entirety and forcing your body to pump out a cascade of anabolic hormones, most notably, growth hormone and testosterone.

Remember, fast-twitch fibers are the largest and have the most potential for growth. So, yes, this program can be used effectively by the off-season bodybuilder, and will result in staggering muscle growth. How many bodybuilders have trained both the speed and high-force components of the fast-twitch fibers? We use both; as long as your nutrition is dialed in, you will grow.

This training program is three days a week. You will be doing three days of intense contrast sets, and we will also give three optional days. You can do one of these optional days, two of them, or all three. But, remember, the primary intended effects are on the three mandatory training days.

Now it's time to take your performance to the next level with the Speed Strong program, while adding slabs of functional muscle in the process. So, whether it's owning the beach with your proudly earned physique at a summertime

Sprinting means all-out, 100 percent full speed. The difference between 90 and 100 percent is everything—akin to the difference between an Ivy League fraternity shoving match with some dude named Thurston and a San Quentin knife fight with the legendary edged weapons expert Don Pentecost.

Keep the following points in mind before sprinting:

1. Raise your body temperature.

Literally warm yourself up a bit. This could be a general warm-up walk, a few minutes on a bike, or even a really light jog. Just get warm. General warm-up should last 5 to 10 minutes. Yes, sprinting in cold weather will require extra warm-up; this is why we are releasing this as a summer program! Sprinting in really cold weather requires extra prep—your body is really, really cold, which can increase injury risk.

2. Do a dynamic warm-up.

Do enough dynamic stretching that you feel energized and ready to go. Stop short of doing so much that you provoke fatigue. If you don't have a go-to dynamic stretch routine, go to the Jailhouse Strong YouTube channel and watch one of our dynamic warm-up routines.

3. Do a few trial ramp-up runs.

Run several moderate-intensity sprints before the work sets begin. Start at about 50 percent max speed and steadily increase it until you hit 90 percent in the last one. This is not an exact science; just work up to near-full speed. And, if you don't feel comfortable hitting full speed because of safety, do the first few weeks of sprints at 90 percent of max speed.

4. Choose the right surface.

In general, natural surfaces are better for sprinting than man-made ones. For example, running on natural grass results in lighter loading on the rear and forefoot, while sprinting on cement places considerably more stress on the rear and forefoot. We recommend sprinting on grass or in sand, if possible. PLEASE AVOID CONCRETE. This program is designed for flat ground. But, if you are prone to hamstring or groin injuries, you can execute these sprints up a hill.

5. If possible, avoid treadmills.

Admittedly, we have used treadmills, but we recommend avoiding them because of danger. Treadmills change the kinematics of the hamstring and exacerbate the risk of hamstring injury, not to mention the risk of getting thrown off the back.

Weightlifting Intensity Levels

When you read over the program, you will notice that some of the weights and reps are listed as RPE with a corresponding number. **RPE,** in strength training, is the **rate of perceived exertion**; it's a subjective measurement of the difficulty of a set.

The RPE scale was introduced to the world decades ago by a Swedish researcher, the late Gunnar Borg, as a measurement of fatigue on a scale of 6 to 20.

Since then, powerlifters like Mike Tuchscherer and others have used RPEs with a more simplified scale and as a way to self-regulate intensity. For example, a strength coach may assign athletes training sessions without specific weights or percentages, but just ask them to work up to a corresponding RPE or rate how difficult a set is using an RPE.

There is no standardized RPE scale for strength training; Borg's original was geared more toward endurance activities. Our scale is listed below. When we assign an RPE, it means the following:

RPE	Meaning
4	Light weight for active recovery or mobility
5	Warm-up weight
6	Too light to have a significant training effect
7	Could have performed an additional three to five reps at the end of the set
8	Could have performed two to three additional reps at the end of the set
9	Could have performed one additional rep at the end of the set, maybe two
10	At a max, no additional reps could be performed at the end of the set

For this program always reference this table. We are aware there are many out there!

Why RPE?

First and foremost, most of you have never trained this way. Using the RPE scale will allow you to adjust the load to fit your performance. For example, if you thrive with this training, you can take advantage by doing more weight when applicable, or more reps when applicable. With RPE, you can let it all hang out on a magical training day and still get the most out of a crappy day.

Most RPE programs assign only weights via an RPE; we assign some weights and some rep schemes. Take advantage of every aspect that this methodology has to offer. It's like you're at the best "Meat 'n' Three" in rural Appalachia—why not try the legendary moonshine with your meal?

Assuming that you are not being emotional, the RPEs will allow reflective feedback beyond classifying something as easy/hard or light/heavy. Also, if your one-repetition max is off, this will not ruin the program (like it can with percentage-based ones).

One of the most important concepts we were mentored with, directly from the late, legendary Dr. Fred Hatfield, is the difference between fast gainers and slow gainers.

"Fast gainers" are people who gain size and strength the easiest. For example, fast gainers are often only able to do 4 to 6 reps at 80 percent of their one-rep max on a given day, while lifters who have trouble making gains are able to rep out at around 15 to 20 reps with 80 percent of their max.

Fast gainers will frequently have poor anaerobic strength endurance. This is explainable, in part, by the fact that their muscular structure is probably mostly white muscle fiber, which has fast-twitch/low-oxidative capabilities. Conversely, slow gainers are probably mostly red muscle fiber (slow-twitch/high-oxidative) and therefore may possess greater ability for rapid recovery during a set.

We can combat this by assigning 80 percent for an RPE of 9. A fast gainer might get five reps, a slow gainer 15 reps, yet both got the desired training results through adaptation. If you are familiar with our past work, we include things like AMRAPs and rest-pause sets to be inclusive to all types of lifters. No one is left out in the cold. Everyone is getting a ticket to the "Gain Train!" So it's time to get on board.

RPE Cautions

Self-awareness is lacking in today's society. Scroll through social media if you want to take a stroll down Delusions of Grandeur Avenue, and swipe left if you want to see Self-Doubt Street.

RPEs are NOT EMOTIONAL. RPEs are not about motivation. They are not about proving your high school coach wrong. RPEs require an honest assessment. If your ego is involved, they will not work.

On the flip side, if you are someone who's always under-valuing yourself or training like a "poodle dick," you will never maximize gains with RPEs!

Make sure you are technically sound in the lifts you are executing. RPEs only work if you are familiar with, and have proper execution of, the assigned movement.

Remember: RPEs require honest self-assessment. If you are unable to do this, find another program!

Fast/Slow Gainer Adjustments

Most people who train seriously are more to the faster gainer side. It is human nature to engage in activities toward which one has a natural propensity. Even weightlifting "hard gainers" are oftentimes really easy gainers, compared to the public at large.

If you are a hard gainer, someone who does 15 reps or more at 80 percent of your one-rep max, you can make the following adjustments:

- Skip days 2 and 4, and do this program over 5 days.
- Extend the prescribed sprint times to 9 to 10 seconds.
- Decrease the rest intervals by 50 percent.

- Increase RPE by 1, so a 7 becomes an 8.
- Add one or two additional series equal to the heaviest ones.

For the fast gainers, those of you doing six reps or fewer at 80 percent of your one-rep max, you can make the following adjustments:

- Extend the work week to 9 days (add extra rest or activity recovery days).
- Shorten the sprints to 4 to 5 seconds.
- Increase rest periods to 240 to 300 seconds.

Bottom line? Most of you will not fall into either extreme camp and should complete the program as prescribed.

Set #2	Exercise	Weight	Reps	Rest Interval	Notes
	Farmer's Walk	85% of deadlift 1RM	50 feet straight	90-180 sec	
	Sprint	Bodyweight	6 seconds straight		

- Farmer's walks should be performed without straps, BUT wear straps if grip limits the weight you can use.
- For the first three weeks, use the same weight. For the second three weeks, you can add 5 to 10 pounds weekly, regardless of strength levels.
- Same guidelines for sprints.

Day 2 (Optional)

Ruck walk at a brisk pace for 30 to 45 minutes. For athletes under 200 pounds, walk with a weighted vest of 15 to 30 pounds. For athletes over 200 pounds, walk with a vest of 30 to 50 pounds. The goal is to keep your heart rate between 120 and 145 beats per minute. If you are in great condition, this might require a very brisk walk going up and down hills; for others, this might require slowing the walk down. If you are unable to ruck for 30 minutes, this program is too intense for you.

Day 3
Series 1 (Bench Press/Plyo Push-Up)

Set #1	Exercise	Weight	Reps	Rest Interval	Notes
	Bench Press	80% of 1RM	RPE 8	75-150 sec	
	Plyometric Push-Ups	Bodyweight	5		

Set #2	Exercise	Weight	Reps	Rest Interval	Notes
	Bench Press	85% of 1RM	RPE 9	75-150 sec	
	Plyometric Push-Ups	Bodyweight	5		

Set #3	Exercise	Weight	Reps	Rest Interval	Notes
	Bench Press	90% of 1RM	RPE 9	75-150 sec	
	Plyometric Push-Ups	Bodyweight	5		

Set #4	Exercise	Weight	Reps	Rest Interval	Notes
	Bench Press	70% of 1RM	RPE 9	75-150 sec	
	Plyometric Push-Ups	Bodyweight	5		

- Any bench press variation is acceptable—incline, decline, flat, dumbbell, even dips are okay.
- For plyometric push-ups, push yourself as high as possible in the air!
- If plyometric push-ups cause pain, med ball chest passes or Smith machine bench press throws are an acceptable substitution for five reps.

Series 2 (Pull-Up/Plyo Pull-Up)

Set #1	Exercise	Weight	Reps	Rest Interval	Notes
	Pull-Ups	BW	RPE 7	75-150 sec	
	Plyometric Pull-Ups	Bodyweight	3		

Set #2	Exercise	Weight	Reps	Rest Interval	Notes
	Pull-Ups	Heavy as possible	5	75-150 sec	
	Plyometric Pull-Ups	Bodyweight	3		

Set #3	Exercise	Weight	Reps	Rest Interval	Notes
	Pull-Ups	Heavy as possible	3	75-150 sec	
	Plyometric Pull-Ups	Bodyweight	3		

Set #4	Exercise	Weight	Reps	Rest Interval	Notes
	Pull-Ups	Heavy as possible	3	75-150 sec	
	Plyometric Pull-Ups	Bodyweight	3		

- Pull-ups: We recommend a neutral grip, but towel pull-up, supinated chin-up, or pronated is acceptable.
- Each week you will go as heavy as possible, so let it hang.
- For the plyo pull-ups, perform the pull-up with enough explosiveness to get air, letting your hands come about an inch off of the bar. Catch the bar with bent elbows, lower into the hang position of your pull-up, and repeat.
- Plyo pull-ups are preferred, but if you are unable to do them, do overhead med ball throws against a wall, throwing from the lats and keeping your arms long.

Day 4 (Optional)

Ruck walk at a brisk pace for 30 to 45 minutes. For athletes under 200 pounds, walk with a weighted vest of 15 to 30 pounds. For athletes over 200 pounds, walk with a vest of 30 to 50 pounds. The goal is to keep your heart rate between 120 and 145 bpm. If you are in great condition, this might require a very brisk walk going up and down hills; for others, this might require slowing the walk down. If you are unable to ruck for 30 minutes, this program is too intense for you.

Day 5
Series 1 (Drop Lunge/Sprint)

Set #1	Exercise	Weight	Reps	Rest Interval	Notes
	Drop Lunges	RPE 7	4 each leg	75-150 sec	2- to 3-inch drop
	Sprint	Bodyweight	6 seconds straight		

Set #2	Exercise	Weight	Reps	Rest Interval	Notes
	Drop Lunges	RPE 8	4 each leg	75-150 Sec	2- to 3-inch drop
	Sprint	Bodyweight	6 seconds straight		

Set #3	Exercise	Weight	Reps	Rest Interval	Notes
	Drop Lunges	RPE 9	4 each leg	75-150 sec	2- to 3-inch drop
	Sprint	Bodyweight	6 seconds straight		

Set #4	Exercise	Weight	Reps	Rest Interval	Notes
	Drop Lunges	RPE 9	4 each leg	75-150 sec	2- to 3-inch drop
	Sprint	Bodyweight	6 seconds straight		

- Drop lunges can be performed with a barbell, specialty bar, or dumbbells, but like all exercises in this program, keep them the same for the entire six weeks. Focus on range of motion and staying true to the RPE; do not sacrifice ROM for weight.

Series 2 (Pendlay Row/Vertical Jump)

Set #1	Exercise	Weight	Reps	Rest Interval	Notes
	Pendlay Rows	RPE 7	5	75-150 sec	
	Vertical Jumps	Bodyweight	5		

Set #2	Exercise	Weight	Reps	Rest Interval	Notes
	Pendlay Rows	RPE 8	5	75-150 sec	
	Vertical Jumps	Bodyweight	5